FATIGUE RECOVERY

Burnout and Compassion Fatigue Prevention Techniques

(The Step-by-step Healing Companion Guide)

Jack Marks

Published by Oliver Leish

Jack Marks

All Rights Reserved

Fatigue Recovery: Burnout and Compassion Fatigue Prevention Techniques (The Step-by-step Healing Companion Guide)

ISBN 978-1-77485-188-3

All rights reserved. No part of this guide may be reproduced in any form without permission in writing from the publisher except in the case of brief quotations embodied in critical articles or reviews.

Legal & Disclaimer

The information contained in this book is not designed to replace or take the place of any form of medicine or professional medical advice. The information in this book has been provided for educational and entertainment purposes only.

The information contained in this book has been compiled from sources deemed reliable, and it is accurate to the best of the Author's knowledge; however, the Author cannot guarantee its accuracy and validity and cannot be held liable for any errors or omissions. Changes are periodically made to this book. You must consult your doctor or get professional medical advice before using any of the suggested remedies, techniques, or information in this book.

Upon using the information contained in this book, you agree to hold harmless the Author from and against any damages, costs, and expenses, including any legal fees potentially resulting from the application of any of the information provided by this guide. This disclaimer applies to any damages or injury caused by the use and application, whether directly or indirectly, of any advice or information presented, whether for breach of contract, tort, negligence, personal injury, criminal intent, or under any other cause of action.

You agree to accept all risks of using the information presented inside this book. You need to consult a professional medical practitioner in order to ensure you are both able and healthy enough to participate in this program.

Table of Contents

INTRODUCTION 1

CHAPTER 1: PAIN MANAGEMENT IN A MEDICAL CONTEXT 3

CHAPTER 2: DETOXIFY YOUR BODY AND EAT HEALTHY FOODS 6

CHAPTER 3: CLASSIFICATION OF THE CONDITION 10

CHAPTER 4: WHAT IS FATIGUE? 15

CHAPTER 5: HOW SLEEP DEPRIVATION AFFECTS YOUR HEALTH 19

CHAPTER 6: WHAT CAN GO WRONG IF YOU HAVE HYPOTHYROIDISM 24

CHAPTER 8: ORGANISE YOUR LIFE 27

CHAPTER 9: MANAGING THE SYMPTOMS 34

CHAPTER 10: ACUPRESSURE 42

CHAPTER 11: KICKING THE BLUES 45

CHAPTER 12: FIRST STEP: DIAGNOSING FIBROMYALGIA .. 51

CHAPTER 13: WHAT ARE THE PSYCHOLOGICAL CAUSES OF FATIGUE? 56

CHAPTER 14: THE SAUNA PROGRAM............................... 58

CHAPTER 15: THE GIVING ELEMENTS............................. 71

CHAPTER 16: STRESS RELIEF 76

CHAPTER 17: HOW TO DEAL WITH STRESS AT WORK 84

CHAPTER 18: NATURALLY BOOSTING TESTOSTERONE..... 89

CHAPTER 19: THE 5 STAGES OF SLEEP............................. 96

CHAPTER 20: SUPPLEMENTS THAT REALLY WORK......... 107

CHAPTER 21: SWAP YOUR JOE FOR A CUP O' GREEN TEA 115

CHAPTER 22: 7 THINGS YOU CAN DO TO GET RID OF FATIGUE 122

CHAPTER 23: WHY IS IT RAW?...................................... 125

CONCLUSION... 131

Introduction

Sometimes fatigue can be a result of something you've done. Sometimes, fatigue can cause you to feel drained and unable to do the things you love. You feel tired and unable to keep up with life's pace. This book is for people who are looking to feel more energetic and to rid themselves of the terrible fatigue that's dragging them down.

This book will explain how tiredness can have entered your life through your actions and your inactions. Although you might feel like you don't have enough energy, energy produces energy. All you have to do is learn how to tap into these resources. This book will show you how. You can also feel more energetic and have more energy by doing a variety of mental and physical exercises. Several friends have experienced this method and were shocked by the quick results.

My method works well for me and my friends, so I knew there would be others who need to get energy back. This is why I wrote this book. You will feel more energetic if you follow the steps in the book.

Follow me as I lead you through these pages of discovery. You'll find that your energy levels increase with each passing moment. This book is your guide to generating energy. It can be very quick to get you on the right track for the time it takes.

Chapter 1: Pain Management in a Medical Context

There are many ways that pain management can be done when someone visits a hospital. The treatment of pain can include medication, such as aspirin or Ibuprofen, surgery, which is more common for more serious injuries, like gunshots and burns, or alternative treatments like hypnosis or massage therapy, or a combination.

The source of pain, side effects, health of the patient, and level of discomfort felt by the patient will all influence the type of medication that is prescribed.

Medication: Different types of medication can be given to patients depending on the situation.

Non-Opioid analgesics – This includes naproxen, ibuprofen and acetaminophen. They can be used to relieve pain and act directly on the area. An enzyme is released when tissue is damaged and produces local pain. This medication stops the release of enzymes and soothes pain. It also reduces inflammation. However, this type of analgesic can cause liver and kidney damage, as well as gastrointestinal discomfort and internal bleeding if used for a prolonged period.

Opioid analgesics – This medication is used to treat higher and more severe levels of pain. They activate the downward pathways of signals by activating synaptic neurons. They bind to Opioid receptors and target different parts of the central nervous system. These include codeine, morphine and meripidine as well as fentanyl, propoxyphine and oxycodone. Side effects can become addictive, and it is possible to take too much of these drugs at different times.

Adjuvant Analgesics are pain relievers that can also be used to treat other conditions. They are used to treat neuropathic pain, which is pain that results from damage to the central nerve system. These include tricyclic antidepressants, antiepileptic drugs, and anesthetics.

Surgery: Surgery should always be the last resort. Surgery is required to end pain pathways if all other pain relievers fail to alleviate it. There are two types of surgery: Rhizotomy which removes a portion of the peripheral nerves and Achordotomy which disables the ascending tracts of the spinal cord, preventing pain signal receptors from reaching the medulla.

Alternative Therapy does not require surgery or drugs. This includes chiropracty, massage, hot compress and acupuncture. It also stimulates nerves to release endorphins. Mental control like hypnosis relies on the brain to ease pain.

Chapter 2: Detoxify your body and eat healthy foods

You can reduce exhaustion and have more energy by detoxing and eating healthy food. This is one of the easiest things you can do. These are some things you can do to detoxify and prevent exhaustion.

Eliminate stimulants.

You may feel tired after drinking stimulants like nicotine, coffee, and soda. Although alcohol is not a stimulant it can cause you to feel tired if taken in large quantities. To detoxify your body, you must first get rid of all the junk that you have put in it.

Avoid bad carbs.

Carbohydrate-rich foods are good for you as they provide energy. All types of carbohydrates may not be created equal. While simple carbohydrates such as bread, pasta, white rice, or bread can increase your energy temporarily, these foods are easy to digest and may cause you to experience an energy crash within 1 to 2 hours. Complex carbohydrates such as whole wheat bread, brown rice and whole wheat pasta are better. These foods are more difficult to digest and will keep your energy up for longer periods.

Get lots of water.

Hydration is one of most common causes for fatigue. It is important to drink enough water each day. Water can help detoxify your body by flushing your system. Although the exact amount of water you should drink is still unknown, 8 ounces 8 times per day or the "8 for Eight" method is very popular. It is also easy to remember.

You should eat foods that detoxify your body and mind.

If you feel tired or exhausted, here are some foods you can eat. These foods can help you detoxify your body as well as your mind.

Cabbage – This tasty vegetable cleanses your liver.

Broccoli – This is rich in antioxidants, and it helps cleanse the liver.

Beets - These beets are great for cleansing the body and removing free radicals.

Avocado - Avocado is rich in antioxidants. It is high in vitamin B and rich in folate, niacin and magnesium.

Asparagus: This superfood helps to prevent aging. It cleanses the body, and contains antioxidants.

Garlic - Garlic improves your immune system, and it boosts your energy.

Green tea - Green Tea helps to eliminate free radicals from the body. It can also be used as a substitute for cola.

Lemongrass - Lemongrass is good for the liver and kidneys.

Wheatgrass – Wheatgrass is good for detoxing and increases metabolism.

Avoid caffeine-containing beverages if you want to boost your energy. High sugar foods like cakes and candy are best avoided as they can cause sugar spikes (and subsequent sugar crashes).

Avoid eating large meals or overeating. Slow down and stop eating when you feel full. Pay attention to your eating habits. It is better to eat small meals each day than to binge eat.

Chapter 3: Classification of the Condition

What is CFS exactly? That's the problem. The condition is not defined in a single way. Different groups may have their own definitions. We can choose the ones that are most agreeable to the community.

The definition from the Center for Disease Control and Prevention (CDC) is the first. It is widely accepted and most commonly used in clinical and research purposes. CFS is defined as a condition that has more than three symptoms beyond fatigue. Six to eight symptoms are required (1994 criteria). This is done using the CDC 1988 scoring system (also known as Holmes system). This definition is also known as Fukuda definition.

Another comes from the Oxford criteria. This covers CFS cases without explanation and the subtype post-infectious fatigue syndrome (or PIFS). This is a notable definition because it requires mental fatigue in order to meet the criteria. It also accepts symptoms that may indicate psychiatric problems.

There is also the 2003 Canadian Clinical Working Definition. The 2003 Canadian Clinical Working Definition states that in order to be classified as CFS/ME in a patient, they must exhibit the following symptoms: fatigue, malaise after exertion and pain, along at least two cognitive signs or neurological signs and at least one of the neuroendocrine or autonomic categories. The illness must last at least six months.

CFS research uses these different definitions. These differences may have an impact on the selection of patients to be studied. Research suggests that heterogeneous CFS may have subtypes.

These case descriptions are used by experts to create clinical practice guidelines for improving diagnosis, treatment and management. The CFS/ME guideline of the National Health Service (based in England & Wales) is one example. This guideline was developed by NICE, the National Institute for Health and Clinical Excellence. It was first published in 2007.

Name of the condition

This group of illnesses is most commonly referred to as "chronic fatigue syndrome". The name, however, is controversial as we have already mentioned. It is not clear if there is a common name that can be used to describe the entire group of conditions. CFS is classified by many authorities as metabolic, post-infectious central nervous system disorder, psychiatric immune system disorder, cardiovascular disorder, and a metabolic, post inflammatory, central nervous system disorder. Different disorders can also cause symptoms to manifest in different ways.

CFS has been called many other names around the globe. Some of these names are: benign myalgic and Akureyri diseases, chronic infectious mononucleosis syndrome, chronic fatigue immune disorder syndrome, myalgic myalgic disease, myalgic-encephalitis syndrome, myalgic neuromyelitis syndrome, myalgic/myalgic syndrome, myalgic flu, raphe nucleusencephalopathy syndrome, Tapanui flu or Royal Free disease. The last one is yuppie flu. CFS is a term that many patients prefer to use, such as myalgic or encephalomyelitis. They believe that chronic fatigue syndrome undermines the condition sufficiently to make it not serious, which discourages research.

A 2001 review found that ME symptoms were a distinct condition. This was based on an article by Acheson from 1959. In literature, ME and CFS are often referred to as the same thing. In 1999, a review stated that the Royal Colleges of Physicians, Psychiatrists, and General Practitioners had recommended CFS as an alternative to ME. CFS was widely used in the UK at that time and the group felt that there wasn't a documented condition in the central nervous system or muscles that ME implied. A editorial stated that there was some acceptance of the review, but also criticism from groups and individuals who supported a name change. They claim that the report was biased and that psychiatric voices dominated, with opposing views not being included. A Lancet commentary in 2002 included a note about the most recent report of the "Working Group on CFS/ME" referring to their decision to use "CFS/ME as a compromise." They use both names to show respect for different opinions and acknowledge that there is still no consensus on the correct term.

Chapter 4: What is Fatigue?

Most people give fatigue many different meanings. Fatigue is a feeling of tiredness due to physical or mental exertion. Fatigue is, however, a state of consciousness that describes a variety of afflictions. Fatigue can be associated with mental and/or physical weakness. However, it can vary from general lethargy to a specific, work-induced burning sensation in the muscles. It is often described as exhaustion or lethargy, languidness or languor, lassitude, lassitude, or listlessness. It is true. This is true. Fatigue can cause you to feel tired and weak, making it difficult to do everyday tasks. Physical fatigue is characterized by the inability to perform at a normal level. This is especially noticeable when you do heavy exercise that requires a lot of energy input. Instead, mental fatigue manifests as somnolence (sleepiness). It is the easiest aspect of fatigue to identify as sleepiness. It can be described as a neurobiological need to sleep, which results from physiological wake or sleep drive. It is distinct from fatigue. While sleepiness refers to the desire to go to sleep, fatigue is the body's signal that it needs to stop doing any ongoing activity (physical, mental, or otherwise). Physical and mental fatigues are the first signs that your body is under stress.

Psychological fatigue refers to a lack of energy and a reluctance or inability to complete a task. While the causes of fatigue, sleepiness, and fatigue may be different, the consequences of both are similar. Some include a decrease in mental or physical performance. Feeling fatigued is when one feels so tired that they are unable to do everyday tasks. Every person experiences fatigue differently. It is not possible to expect everyone to feel the same fatigue effects. Sometimes fatigue can be accompanied by pain. Sometimes it can feel like you don't have control over your own life.

Fatigue can be a sign or symptom. Fatigue is not a sign of an illness or a condition. Fatigue is a feeling of being tired, lethargic and lacking energy. You shouldn't conclude that you are tired if you feel tired or less energetic than usual. Fatigue can seriously affect your ability to function and make it difficult for you to manage even the most basic of life's tasks. This can affect your mind and body. Changes in diet, environment, stress levels, and sleep can most often resolve fatigue.

Fatigue can be a sign of a larger problem. You need to assess the factors that contribute to your fatigue. To determine the cause of fatigue, a specialist will perform a medical examination. This is especially important if you feel fatigued and it is becoming more frequent. Chronic Fatigue Syndrome (CFS) is a more severe form of fatigue. Chronic Fatigue Syndrome (CFS) is a chronic fatigue syndrome that can cause severe symptoms such as recurring sore throats and muscle pain.

Chronic fatigue is defined as persistent fatigue that lasts at least six months consecutively. If the threshold is not met, it should not be taken as a sign that someone is suffering from chronic fatigue.

Patterns

Chapter 5: How Sleep Deprivation Affects Your Health

As they need air and food to function properly, our bodies also need sleep. The body begins to heal itself and restore its chemical balance when it goes to sleep. New connections are made in the brain that help memory retention. Your body and brain will not function normally if you don't get enough sleep. This will impact your quality of life. A study found that a sleep schedule of six hours or less increases the chance of death by 12 percent.

These are some clear indicators of sleep deprivation:

Yawning

Irritability;

Sleepiness excessive

Daytime fatigue.

The body cannot be overpowered by stimulants like caffeine or other stimulants. Sleep deprivation can cause serious problems in the body's internal systems. Continue reading to learn about the various effects of sleep deprivation upon different body systems.

The central nervous system

For the proper functioning of the central nervous systems, sleep is essential. Chronic sleeplessness can lead to changes in how information is sent. Your brain's neurons help you retain new memories by getting to sleep. Your brain will become exhausted if you don't get enough sleep. This means that you'll be unable focus or learn new things. You may experience a delay in your body signals, which can reduce coordination and make you more susceptible to accidents.

Lack of sleep can also affect your mental health. This can cause mood swings, and it can also compromise creativity and decision-making. Hallucinations, depression, and other long-term effects can result. It is possible to feel dizzy and weak during the day. This can make driving unsafe.

The immune system

The immune system creates cytokines, which are infection-fighting substances, when we sleep. These substances are used in fighting bacteria and viruses. These substances also promote sleep and provide energy for the immune system to fight illness. Your immune system won't be able to work properly if you don't get enough sleep. It is possible to get sick quickly and take a while to recover.

The respiratory system

Sleep apnea is a condition that can disrupt sleep and lead to sleep deprivation. This can make you more susceptible to common respiratory infections like the flu or the common cold. Chronic lung disease, such as chronic sleep deprivation, can also be worsened by sleep deprivation.

The digestive system

Obesity can be caused by lack of exercise or overeating. Not sleeping enough can also lead to obesity. Ghrelin, a hormone that controls hunger and fullness, can be negatively affected by a lack of sleep. Leptin signals the brain to stop eating. Ghrelin is produced when you aren't sleeping. This stimulates your appetite. If you're not getting enough sleep, you can gain weight. You won't be able to exercise and you may feel tired. You are at greater risk for developing type 2 diabetes if you don't get enough sleep.

The Endocrine System

You need to get enough sleep for hormones to function properly. For testosterone production, you need to get at least three hours sleep each night. Hormone production will be affected if you stay awake at night. Hormones are responsible for building muscle mass and repairing cells.

The Cardiovascular system

Insufficient sleep can disrupt the healthy blood vessels and heart function. This includes blood sugar, blood pressure, and inflammation. Sleeping well is crucial for your body's ability repair blood vessels and heal.

Chapter 6: What can go wrong if you have hypothyroidism

Hypothyroidism may not be a problem in the early stages. However, if it isn't treated, it can lead to very serious illness. Hypothyroidism has been linked to an increased risk of developing heart disease. Low levels of thyroid hormones cause an increase in bad cholesterol. High levels of bad cholesterol can cause a reduction in your heart's ability to pump blood. This can lead to an increase in the size of your heart and ultimately, heart failure.

Hypothyroidism may also cause goiter. This is a condition in which the thyroid gland grows excessively. This is because the body constantly stimulates the thyroid gland to produce more thyroid hormones, which in turn stimulates the thyroid gland to increase its size and causes it to grow. Although it is not dangerous, a goiter can cause problems with swallowing, breathing, and your natural appearance.

Mental illness can also be caused by it. If left untreated, it can lead to severe depression that can get worse over time. It can also lead to a slowing down of brain function.

If Hypothyroidism goes untreated, it can lead to peripheral neuropathy (damage to the peripheral nerves of the body). The body's peripheral nerves are important. These nerves link your brain to your spinal cord and connect to your arms and legs, allowing information to flow throughout your body. When these nerves become damaged, the body may feel pain, numbness, or tingling sensations in the affected areas. This can lead to muscle weakness, and eventually loss of control.

Low levels of thyroid hormones can cause infertility in women, as it interferes in ovulation.

Myxedema is another serious consequence of hypothyroidism. This is a potentially life-threatening condition that can be caused by long-term hypothyroidism. Myxedema coma is easily triggered by infection or stress. Myxedema patients should seek immediate medical attention. It can cause drowsiness and unconsciousness as well as intense cold intolerance.

Untreated hypothyroidism can increase the risk of having babies with birth defects than healthy women. Babies with untreated hypothyroidism are more likely to have serious intellectual or developmental problems. It can also affect the baby's physical development.

If you have read all of the information above, then continue to the next chapter for more information about the treatment options. You will also find information about possible side effects of medical treatments in the next chapter.

Chapter 8: Organise Your Life

Chaos and clutter are two things that can cause fatigue. If you want to feel less tired, organize your house, your workspace, and your entire life. You can do many things to organize your life. These are just a few of the many things you can do to make your life easier.

Create lists

It is easier to list everything so you can remember what you need. It can be exhausting to try and remember everything. Having lists will save you the effort of remembering and memorizing things. You should make a list before you go grocery shopping. You should also make a list of what you need to do the next day at the end of each day. To make sure you have a budget, it is important to list all of your monthly expenses. A list of people you want to send Christmas cards or purchase gifts to can be created. Your lists can be written in a notebook or organizer, or you can use your smartphone or laptop to create them.

Make a schedule and set deadlines

It is also important to set deadlines and create schedules for everything you have to do. This will help you to avoid wasting time and allow you to relax. You will feel overwhelmed if you don't know how to manage your time. You can stay focused by creating a timeline and a deadline. Be realistic about setting deadlines and scheduling. Don't be too strict when setting deadlines. You will feel more stressed and tired if your deadline is too strict.

Don't procrastinate

Procrastinating will only make your work more difficult. You will be more stressed if you procrastinate, as you must rush to meet the deadline. You also get poor quality output. You can start your tasks early so you don't have to rush. You can also stop worrying about the task and relax by completing it early. If you complete your tasks before the deadline, it will feel like a weight has been lifted from your shoulders.

You must stick to your schedule when you set deadlines and create a calendar. Instead of getting distracted by checking your email or checking social media, you should be able to focus on the task at hand and not get distracted.

How to Prioritize

People can become overwhelmed by the sheer number of tasks they have to complete in a given day. Remember that you don't have superpowers, and can only complete one task at a given time. To avoid feeling exhausted after completing all of your tasks, you need to learn how to prioritize. If you have a long list of tasks to complete, such as shopping for Christmas gifts, and it is March, you will feel overwhelmed and exhausted. You can put off Christmas shopping, and other tasks that you don't really need right now. These tasks should be completed only after you have finished with all other tasks.

Declutter your home

If you want to be able to relax and unwind in your home, you should start decluttering it. It will be easier to relax and unwind if your home is clean and well-organized. Your house will make you feel more stressed and fatigued, which can lead to further fatigue. Get rid of clutter in your home now.

You must dispose of any items that you don't use or like, such as old clothes, DVDs, books, and toys. They can be given away or sold at a yard sales. Also, you should throw away any broken items that are not repairable. Only keep the things you use. You should have plenty of storage units such as shelves, drawers, cabinets, so that you don't clutter up your home. You can reduce clutter in your home by giving everything a place to call home.

Avoid buying items at sales or bargain prices unless absolutely necessary. People have a tendency to purchase things that they don't need or want simply because the price has been reduced by 50% or more. You should always consider whether you actually need the item before you purchase it at a discount price. Be honest about your answer.

De-clutter your workspace

De-cluttering your workspace is another important tip for organizing your life. You will be more productive if you get rid of clutter in your work area. Clear your desk regularly. Don't leave documents and files piled up on your desk. A tray should be provided for all incoming and outgoing documents. A file cabinet is a good choice for all the documents you don't need right away but will be useful for later. A drawer divider can be installed to organize office supplies such as paperclips and staples, pencils and pencils. You will find it easier to work when everything is in the right place.

Delegate tasks

Delegating tasks is another way to reduce fatigue. You don't have to do everything yourself. You should properly delegate tasks to subordinates if you are a supervisor or manager. You can ask your children and other household members to assist you in the chores at home. You must take responsibility for your actions and not rely on others.

Learn how to say "no"

You need to be aware of your limitations mentally and physically in order to prevent fatigue. If you feel unable to handle additional tasks or responsibilities, you should learn to say "no". You shouldn't work overtime every time your boss asks you to. Pay attention to your body, and learn how you can decline. You can politely decline to go out with friends and drink alcohol on Friday nights. However, it is a sign that you are not interested in going out with your friends after work.

Chapter 9: Managing the Symptoms

Chronic fatigue syndrome is often treated with medications that only manage its symptoms.

PAIN KILLERS are used to relieve joint pains and sore muscles. The use of anti-inflammatory drugs can also relieve severe pain, headaches, and frequent fevers. If the painkiller does not work, consult your doctor immediately. Naproxen, ibuprofen, and acetaminophen are the most commonly prescribed over-the-counter medications. These drugs can be used to relieve severe or persistent muscle and joint pains, fevers, and headaches. Follow the doctor's instructions and read the label carefully.

ANTISEIZURE/ANTICONVULSANTS- are the type of prescription drugs such as pregabalin and gabapentin that are usually prescribed for sleep difficulties and pain.

NARCOTICS- can be prescribed when pain cannot be managed with other over-the-counter medications. This is often used for severe cases such as chronic fatigue syndrome. To avoid becoming addicted, this can only be used for a short time.

ANTIDEPRESSANTS- Helps to reduce anxiety and depression, improve sleep quality and concentration. It helps prevent the development of depression, which is a common side effect in those with this condition. Chronic fatigue syndrome can make the patient's situation worse. Therefore, it is important to treat this condition.

Although there have been studies that corticosteroids are effective in treating chronic fatigue syndrome (CFS), there are other researches that show that they don't work well for treating CFS. It can also cause serious side effects.

Quality Life and Sleep Management

Fatigue can be made worse by any changes in the patient's sleep pattern. The condition can be affected by too much or too little sleep. Persons with CFS should avoid sleeping during the day. To help the body adapt, any changes should be made gradually.

Get enough rest

Rest is more important than actual sleep. It is important to gradually introduce rest periods into the patient's daily life. A 30-minute break is ideal.

Relaxation

Relaxation can be very beneficial as it improves sleep quality and reduces stress, anxiety, and pain. Some relaxation techniques, such as meditation and breathing techniques, can be useful during rest periods.

Proper diet

A balanced diet is important for alleviating symptoms, just as with any other condition. Avoid food and drinks that are allergic to you. Reduce the amount of food you eat and eat meals that are high in essential nutrients.

CFS and sleep dysfunction

Chronic fatigue syndrome patients often have a variety of symptoms and severity. These symptoms can be disruptive and disabling, so it is important that the doctor and patient communicate to find a way to manage the condition. Most cases of severe symptoms can be treated directly.

Studies show that patients suffering from chronic fatigue syndrome have sleep problems. Patients with chronic fatigue syndrome often complain of difficulty sleeping, frequent awakenings, vivid dreams, insomnia, hypersomnia, extreme sleepiness, and night-time sleep spasms. Patients feel more tired and less refreshed after a night of sleep.

Doctors help patients get quality sleep by encouraging them to adopt healthy sleeping habits. They also taught sleep hygiene practices and sleep techniques that promote sleep.

To establish a routine, try to go to bed every night.

- Avoid naps during daytime.

- Don't work, watch TV, or eat in your bed. It should be solely for rest and sleep.

Control the temperature, light and noise in your bedroom.

Avoid alcohol, caffeine, and tobacco.

A 30-minute walk or light exercise early in the morning can improve your sleep quality.

If these methods fail to work, your doctor may recommend antihistamines and sleeping pills as the initial treatment. If the patient continues to feel "unrefreshed" after each sleep, they may want to consult a sleep specialist in order to evaluate the situation further.

Handling Pain

CFS patients often experience severe pain in the joints and muscles. Chronic fatigue syndromes sufferers often complain of headaches and skin soreness.

Most doctors will recommend prescription and over-the counter pain relief. Others would recommend pain therapy. Experts recommend that people who experience constant pain seek counselling and other techniques to manage their pain. These include stretching, heat, gentle massage, heating, toning exercises and relaxations techniques, as well as movement therapies. If done by a qualified practitioner, alternative methods like acupuncture may also be used to relieve pain.

Complaints about memory and concentration

These are the most severe symptoms of chronic fatigue syndrome. There are many ways to help the patient with chronic fatigue syndrome. These include meditation and relaxation techniques, memory aids such as planners, organizers, and resource manuals. The patient should also try to stimulate their mind with crosswords, puzzles, and other board games.

Patients should be cautious when taking stimulants that are prescribed for cognitive problems. Some stimulants can cause a push-crash and relapses.

Combat Depression

Chronic fatigue syndrome is often associated with depression. This is because the patient must adjust to a weakening or undermining illness. Nearly half of chronic fatigue syndrome patients develop depression, which can exacerbate other symptoms. Although CFS cannot be cured, treatment can reduce stress and anxiety.

If the correct dosage and variant of anti-depressant medication is used, it can be helpful. Anti-depressants can cause side effects that may be worsening the condition. Screening tools are available to help identify any psychological disorders or depression. Deep breathing, muscle relaxations practices, tai-chi, and yoga are all beneficial to some patients. These activities promote a sense of well-being and help to reduce anxiety.

Chapter 10: Acupressure

Traditional Chinese Medicine states that acupuncture and Acupressure are based upon the theory of the meridians. Meridians are energy pathways through the body. To address problems in the stomach or abdomen, acupuncture and acupressure can be used on our feet and hands.

Back of the hand - This is the point where the thumb and index fingers meet at the back side of the hand. It has been proven to relieve headaches, colds and constipation. Gently rub it with the opposite hand. Both hands should be used for the acupressure. This should be avoided by pregnant women.

Wrist – The area running from the thumb to your wrist is the one you need to be watching. To relieve headaches, dizziness, sore throat, cough, stiff neck, stiff neck, stiffness, and sore throat, rub the area gently. Interlock your thumbs and allow the index finger to massage the wrist. This is exactly what you need to be watching out for. Repeat the massage with your other hand. It is best to do this for between 2 and 5 minutes each day.

Acupressure on your ear can help reduce your appetite. This is important for those who want to lose weight or keep their weight off. The small, tiny flap is located in front of you. The flap should be held so that your fingers reach the front and back of the small flap. For approximately one minute, press the points onto your ears. This can be done when you are feeling very hungry, or before you eat your meal. This will help you to control your portion sizes and decrease your appetite. This will allow you to lose weight.

Leg - This acupressure treatment can be used if you want to lose weight, or if you have digestive problems such as vomiting, stomachache, diarrhea, and distention. You should pay attention to the area below your knee. Place your three first fingers below your knee. Look out for a slight depression as your middle finger moves towards your leg. For immediate relief, you can gently massage the area. Do this 2 to 3 times per day. This will give you relief.

Head - The area where the skull bones meet at the back of the head is where a small depression. Look out with your hand for the depression. For relief from sleep-related disorders and insomnia, gently press this point. This should be done for approximately 10 minutes each night, just before you go to bed. You may also find that acupressure can improve your quality of sleep.

Chapter 11: Kicking the Blues
ORGANIC COCONUT OIL

Coconut oil is often mentioned by those who have been involved in the real food movement or watched Dr. Oz. Coconut oil was once a stigmatized product because of its high saturated fat content. However, it appears that coconut oil is finally making a comeback in mainstream health care.

Coconut oil is the richest part of coconut. Coconut oil is stable at room temperature, much like butter. It does not become rancid in heat, light, or in heat like other oils. I think it has a lovely tropical scent.

It can be a great way to increase your intake of healthy fats and it is also helpful in the assimilation fat-soluble vitamins.

Coconut oil was once a part of "health" advice that advised against saturated fats for years.

Coconut oil is an amazing oil that can be used in many ways. You can use it in smoothies, yogurt, oatmeal, and even on your skin to moisturize. Coconut oil is rich in medium-chain saturated fats (MCFAs), which are a healthier form of saturated fat than trans-fat. Consuming trans-fatty acids is associated with increased cholesterol, depression, and heart disease. What about coconut oil containing MCFA fats? These fats are quickly metabolized in the liver and converted into energy. Yes.

WHEATGRASS SHOTS

Wheatgrass is a type of wheatgrass that is rich in nutrients. It can be purchased in powder or liquid form as a dietary supplement. Wheatgrass can be used to make juicing or as a flavoring for smoothies and tea.

Wheatgrass contains a high level of nutrients including iron, calcium, magnesium, amino acids, chlorophyll, vitamins A and C, as well as vitamins A and E. Wheatgrass is touted as a treatment for anemia, diabetes and constipation. It also helps with skin conditions, cancer, arthritis, joint pain, and balancing sugar.

You can drink it as a 1-ounce fresh juice. Wheatgrass powders can be purchased at your local health food store if this option is not possible. This $2.00 shot will be your best, and you can still drive.

Becky shared some great information about wheatgrass in (FOREVER YOUNG), a blog I am a part of.

"Many years ago, a woman instilled a new way of healing that has been an effective path for many. Ann Wigmore learned natural healing secrets from her grandmother in Lithuania. Ann discovered the healing properties of wheatgrass after her grandmother, who used greens and other moss poultices to heal wounded soldiers during WWI.

Ann, 18, broke her legs at the ankles in an accident. Gangrene set in. The well-meaning doctors in the early 1900's planned to amputate. Ann, relying on the wisdom of her grandmother, refused to have her legs amputated and instead placed herself on the hospital's lawn each day, to absorb the sun's healing rays. Ann ate grass from her chair, and her uncle brought her edible flowers. Ann was contacted by a doctor who asked to take a tissue sample for his laboratory. This is an incredible and almost unbelievable twist. Ann was able to use both her legs for the rest, thanks to the amazing results.

Ann later discovered that sprouted wheatberry grass was superior to all other grasses. This finding led to Ann starting a few clinics that offer grass therapy. It is used today to reverse cancers, tumors, and other 'incurables'. After learning the wheatgrass diet and the living foods diet, people who have been through conventional chemotherapy and other treatments find that they no longer fear the possibility of having their condition recur.

Ann Wigmore established clinics in San Fidel (NM), Puerto Rico, Palm Beach (FL), Lemon Grove, CA, and a new one in Virginia.

Visit: www.wigmore.org www.optimumhealth.org

EMF - BLUES

You are probably carrying a digital device if you're like most people in western countries. You have a cell phone, tablet, notebook, laptop and kindle. All of them carry electromagnetic frequencies, also known as EMF's.

EMF's can make you feel weaker, particularly after working all day on your computer. Even talking on your cell phone for long periods of time can leave you feeling tired. EMFs can disrupt your natural flow. Walking near trees, a waterfall, or in an outdoor café or garden can lift your mood and make you feel more alive and vibrant.

There are a few high-quality technology devices available that can help you balance and harmonize the bio-energy system of your body, which will allow it to perform at its best.

EFORCE PLUS offers bracelets and pendants for both men and women. They look just like jewelry, but the technology is hidden on the other side. These products have been shared with me and my friends by clients and friends, as I noticed a difference in how I felt about four years ago when I began using them. Clients and friends told me they feel refreshed after long days of working around electronic gadgets.

Electronic devices will be around for a long time, so we are m

We should do everything we can to protect our bodies.

Chapter 12: First Step: Diagnosing Fibromyalgia

Chronic fatigue syndrome (or Fibromyalgia) can cause you to feel tired and irritable. Both chronic diseases can cause severe pain and affect quality of life. Although these conditions have specific criteria, they are often overlooked because of the normal blood tests. The distinction between these syndromes is also not clear.

Fibromyalgia can't be diagnosed by a simple blood test or X-ray. A physical exam is required to determine the diagnosis. The history of the patient must also be taken into consideration. To rule out other diseases such as Fibromyalgia, doctors can still order x-rays or blood tests.

Tender Points

According to the American College of Rheumatology (ACR), the patient must have pain for at least three months before the diagnosis can be made. Muscle pain must also be felt at specific areas of the body, also known as tender points. The back and neck are the most sensitive areas with 18 points.

Routine lab tests are not able to reveal Fibromyalgia's widespread pain. Physical examinations of pressure points are used to diagnose Fibromyalgia. Fibromyalgia patients feel pain in their muscles, even when the least pressure is applied to them, especially at their tender points. A physical exam will confirm if there is pain or discomfort at any of these tender points.

The patient must have experienced widespread pain (four quadrants) in her body for at least three consecutive months to meet the criteria. The patient must also feel light pressure at 11 of the 18 tender points. Many chronic pain syndromes mirror the Fibromyalgia. The American College of Rheumatology has identified the disease's criteria as being 88% accurate.

Tender points vs. trigger points

There is a distinction between tender points and trigger points. Trigger points can be described as nodules you feel in your muscles that look like ropes. The trigger points can be pressed to cause pain in the affected area. However, if tender points are present, it will only cause discomfort in the area. This is good news, as it opens up the door to other treatments. There are many treatments that can be used to relieve painful knots. Studies have shown that relieving pain from a single trigger point can significantly reduce the severity of the general pain. The therapeutic massage is one of the most popular methods to do this. The therapeutic massage works by relaxing the muscles and removing trigger points. Hot showers, as well as a quick soak in the hot tub, can help reduce trigger points and ease muscle tension. Trigger points can also cause tightness in the muscles that will eventually spread to other areas of the body.

A diagnosis can still be applied to a person if they do not meet the requirements of possessing 11 of the 18 tender points. They can also follow other guidelines that are less restrictive. A group of rheumatologists, working for ACR, had developed new criteria that doctors must use to diagnose Fibromyalgia. This new criteria has its pros and cons. It can be used to replace the tender point's criteria with a checklist of symptoms.

The symptoms and effects of Fibromyalgia can be overwhelming and frustrating, especially if the patient doesn't have the right knowledge to manage the condition. Fibromyalgia can be greatly eased by group support from family, friends, communities, and other organizations.

Numerous studies have also shown that stressors, such as environmental, emotional, and physical, can help relieve symptoms. It is important to consult a Fibromyalgia specialist or practitioner who is familiar with the subject.

Could it be Chronic Fatigue Syndrome (CFS)?

To determine whether the disease is easy or requires early treatment, doctors will usually order that the patient undergo tests. The doctor will consider diagnosing the patient if there is nothing seriously wrong with the results.

It is important to recognize that symptoms of this disease are very similar to those of other chronic diseases such as chemicals sensitivities and myofascial syndrome. It is difficult to diagnose this disease because of the many symptoms and disorders. Therefore, it is better to treat the symptoms than seek a diagnosis.

Chapter 13: What are the Psychological Causes of Fatigue?

Your level of power can drop if you are tired, stressed, anxious, frustrated, or exhausted. Are you going through a major event like a shift, a separation, or a new job recently? These events can be stressful both mentally and physically.

This is a condition that can only be treated if the cause is clear. These problems have been treated before. However, if the symptoms persist for more than two weeks, you should consult a psychologist.

Get a Physician

If you are not getting the necessary rest, nourishment and emotional support, it is wise to visit the doctor. Exhaustion can indicate a problem in your healthcare.

Your medical center lists several health issues that could cause exhaustion, including anemia (iron deficiencies), cardiovascular disease, diabetes, thyroid problems and other conditions. You could also be exhausted by allergic reactions, a lack of supplement D, or medications you are taking.

Your doctor will perform a complete checkup and do bloodwork to determine the root cause of your problems and suggest ways you can correct them.

Your doctor may be able to help you understand the cause of your exhaustion by looking at how it looks. If you wake up in the morning feeling relaxed, but then feel exhausted quickly, this could be a sign of an underactive hypothyroid. You may also feel frustrated if your energy levels drop and you experience exhaustion throughout the day.

Don't be alarmed if all this makes you feel anxious. According to the institution, exhaustion is not a sign of serious illness and is often a common sign. Make sure to schedule a check-up.

Chapter 14: The Sauna Program

You may sauna if you are a CBS Upregulator.

Eliminate glutathione. Saunas can be used even if you have an EMF sensitivity. To do this, heat the sauna before using it and then unplug the unit.

There are many types of saunas available today. The most popular saunas today are far infrared, high dry heat, and ozone. Fred Nelson provided me with a high-heat cloth sauna. (No longer available). It is no more available. William Rea, M.D., was my first doctor. My doctor. I wouldn't recommend using a sauna that isn't outgassed if you have a chemical reaction to wood. 18 years ago, I was unable to safely enter any wooden sauna other than the tiled sauna at Dr. Reas' clinic or my cloth sauna.

Rule of thumb...

A weekly fasting blood test may be necessary if you sauna more than three times per week. A prescription can be obtained from your doctor. You can then take it to the nearest laboratory.

Low ferritin levels are common in chemically sensitive people. My ferritin was 2 and Dr. Rea advised me to sauna. It should be at least 15. However, if you are extremely sick or malnourished and have a ferritin of 15, it is a good idea to have it above 15. A lot of women have ferritin levels between 6-12.

Take a multivitamin/multi-mineral with iron if your ferritin levels are low. Dr. Rea advised me to sauna even though I couldn't tolerate iron. You can do what you want.

Others suggest that you cook in a cast-iron pan to make iron. This is what I do. The iron supplement is not required for post-menopausal women and men.

If you feel uncomfortable or woozy while in the sauna, "Get out!"

Eat at least an hour before you start the sauna. You might vomit if you have a large breakfast and then go to the sauna. Prescription medications should be taken after the sauna to ensure that you don't get irritated.

The goal of your sauna therapy is to get the body to sweat.

About 20% of the toxins in your skin will be eliminated through sweating or outgassing. Around 80% of toxic substances will be eliminated through the liver, kidneys and bladder. They are then deposited into the colon and bladder as urine and fecal matter.

Sauna converts fat-soluble chemicals to water-soluble chemicals, which can be excreted via detox organs like the kidneys, liver and skin.

Individuals will vary in how long they stay in the sauna. One person might stay in the sauna for 10 minutes while another person may stay there for 20 minutes. The length of your sauna session will depend on how healthy you are.

You can try another round if you reach 30 minutes. It is best to wait for several hours before you start a second round of sauna.

Sauna preparation

* Keep track of your weight

* Exercise if you can. Do not exercise if you are suffering from Chronic Fatigue.

* In 6 oz. Add:

* 1/2 teaspoon Tri-salts (Ecological Forms).

* 1/8 teaspoon salt

* 1 teaspoon Magnesium Chloride

* 200 mg. buffered Vitamin C

* 500 mg. Liposomal Galutathione (do NOT take if you are a CBS ++).).

* 1/2 teaspoon Selenium Selenite, ARG or Selenium Methionine. (Whatever you are able to tolerate)

* A Niacin supplement can be taken to vasodilate blood vessels. It was too much for me. Start with 25mgs if you want to give niacin a try.

Temperature Setting

* High Heat: Not more than 150 degrees. Yes, I do know that people can go higher but they don't.

* Infrared can reach as low as 110 degrees

What to wear, and what to bring with you

* A few large glasses each with 12 oz. Clean water for every 15 minutes spent in the sauna. (No plastic bottles).

* You can either sauna naked or in a tee shirt with shorts.

* A small towel or washcloth to remove sweat. Reabsorption is not what we want.

* Towel to use as a seat.

Finding the right balance between downloading and sauna is key. I love this term from computer tech! Chemicals from fat tissue are removed by chelating and extricating them.

After the sauna...

Shower and scrub: After the sauna, you should take a shower. Make sure to use a washcloth for your body.

After Sauna Supplements...

You don't know when it will end, so make sure to take these supplements right after your sauna session.

* 1/2 tsp/ Trisalts dissolved into water

* 1/8 teaspoon salt

* Multivitamin/multi-mineral caps with or without iron.3 Tablespoons of olive oil or coconut oil; or any tolerated oil is OK.

* 1 Tablespoon psyllium

* Measure your weight. If your weight is lower than it was before the sauna, you may be dehydrated. You will need another glass of fluid.

The Process

Please let us know if you feel the need to go slower or faster than what is suggested. Your body is your responsibility. When you try out the new sauna program, remember to "Be Confident." Everything will work out. Your personal best is what you want, not the goals of your friends.

Ozone saunas are a different kind of sauna. Ozone saunas combine steam and ozone. The chamber will extend your head. Ozone is not recommended for people with reactive airways.

It's a smart idea to do some research on ozone saunas and to try them out in the office of a certified practitioner before you buy the equipment. I have not used an ozone sauna since 2010. I found this sauna to be exhilarating. When used properly and in a well ventilated area, ozone doesn't bother my skin. Promolife.com sells a variety of rectal/vaginal Ozone suppositories. You can choose from a variety of base oils.

EXAMPLE A 7-WEEK SAUNA PARTNERSHIP

Your sauna program may last seven weeks or seven weeks, depending on how toxic you are. I was severely emaciated. I was allergic to all foods, and my bones were broken. You will need to take it slow if you're like me. Niacin is not recommended. If you don't feel the need to sweat immediately, do not panic. Most likely, you won't. This is how your sauna schedule might look:

WEEK 1

Day 1: Sauna for 5-10 minutes

Day 2: 10 minutes

Day Three: 10 minutes

Day 4: 15 minutes

Day Five: 15 Minutes

Day Six: 15 Minutes

Day Seven: 15 Minutes

WEEK 2

Day 1: 20 minutes

Day 2: 20 minutes

Day Three: 20 Minutes

Day 4: 20 minutes

Day Five: 20 Minutes

Day Six: 20 Minutes

Day Seven: 20 Minutes

WEEK 3

Increase your sauna time from 5 to 25 minutes each day.

WEEK 4

Increase your sauna time from 5 to 30 minutes each day. It was difficult for me to increase it. For seven weeks, I couldn't get beyond 20 minutes. You can do it again! Do your best.

WEEK 5-7

You can either keep your sauna time at 30 minutes or go for the longest time you are comfortable.

EXAMPLE A SAUNA PROGRAM

FOR A HEALTHIER PERSON

The person who is normal in body weight I call "Healthier". He or she appears to have high levels of toxic chemical in their bodies, even though they are not sick. They might be suffering from chronic fatigue. They might be able to eat a variety of foods.

Here's how your sauna schedule could look if you're looking to be healthier.

You can increase the amount by 25mgs.-75mgs. You can also add niacin to your exercise routine. Your body will experience a flush of redness. Use it if you are able to tolerate it. It dilates blood vessels, which allows for deeper detoxification.

WEEK 1

Day 1: 20 minutes

Day 2: 20 minutes

Day Three: 25 Minutes

Day 4: 30 minutes

Day Five: 30 Minutes

Day Six: 35 Minutes

Day Seven: 35 Minutes

WEEK 2

Two rounds of 30 minute each may be possible.

Day 1: AM 30 minutes, PM 30 minutes

Day 2: AM: 30 mins; PM: 30 mins

Continue on to Day 7

WEEK 3-7

Two 45 minute rounds daily

SAUNA MAINTENANCE SCHEDULE

These schedules are just examples. Your sauna time will be determined by you. After seven weeks of the 7-day sauna detoxification program, you can start a maintenance program. Some people feel the need for a second round of 7-day sauna detoxification after 6 months.

According to some people, there is a barrier that prevents you from entering a sauna. Your body will begin to feel the hot air as cool. That barrier has never been broken. I can't stay in an infrared sauna or high heat for that long.

The amount of sauna required is a matter of debate in the world. Experts agree with L. Ron Hubbard's approach of doing sauna multiple times per day over a time period of weeks. Others recommend sauna only 2-3x weekly. All experts agree that nutrients are vital.

Chemically sensitive women take longer to sweat. It will happen, don't worry.

Chapter 15: The Giving Elements

It's great to help others. It is often possible to do more for someone else than you can for yourself. It is very ingratifying to be able give. You may feel exhausted if you let yourself be used on an ongoing basis. Balance is what you must find. This can be achieved by assessing which things make you happy and which add stress to your daily life. This is done by asking yourself these questions:

* Would you like to do this?

* Does it make you feel better?

* Can you give without any expectation?

* Does it improve my sense of well-being?

If you don't think the thing you are giving is in line with these rules, it could cause stress. You will have more energy and more fun if you do something because you love it. Positive energy drives people to go beyond their limits, and it will make you feel happier. You don't need to worry about it. The problem is that people often give without expectations or strings attached. Stress is a common problem.

* I make sure my daughter has a great education. I want her to be a doctor.

* I volunteer at my local grocery store to help get groceries cheaper

These are just a few examples, but they should be enough to show you the point. If you expect a return, and it doesn't happen, you can feel disappointed and stressed. Many people tell me that they feel stressed because of others. We know this from previous chapters. So what is the problem?

It is impossible to price the things you do. While you might be able to in a work environment, it is not possible in daily life. However, if you want to do good things for others, it must be your natural behavior and not because you expect something in return. You won't find the happy place within you if you seek validation from others. Many people believe that others will behave in a certain manner or validate the actions of those who give. I've seen this happen many times. The giver will feel used and unhappy if there isn't validation. Sometimes they may feel extremely stressed because they don't know what to do wrong. It is important to remember that any positive act of kindness that someone does for another person should not be taken as a reward. It will never be appreciated by the receiver if it comes with a price tag.

Learn to be patient and give without stress

This attitude of giving can be applied in many ways. It will reduce stress and improve your mood. Volunteerism is one of the best ways to bring things in balance. If you can see others who are less fortunate than you, it will likely make you feel better about your situation. You will be more likely to offer your help if you have no expectations. Because you've found the true meaning and value of giving, stress levels will drop. It can be as simple as helping out at a soup kitchen, volunteering in an animal shelter, or simply doing something nice for an elderly neighbor. This shows that you can give without expecting anything in return, which boosts your positive energy. It is important to realize that giving is not about expecting anything in return. Stress can be caused by putting a price tag on the things you do for others. Don't give without strings attached, it will backfire.

You have probably ever felt the pain of being the one who was angry at someone for not reacting in a way they expected. This is how people feel when they give without strings attached. You should give with no expectations and be positive. It will help you feel better about yourself, let go of stress, and make you feel happier. Giving is a way to feel helpful and useful. You will feel great inside if you give for the right reasons. Giving gives you the ability to feel fulfilled. As we have discussed in previous chapters, this is what your life is all about. It is easy to see that the purpose of your existence will be clear if you only give to the right people. You can actually feel good about being there for someone who needed you. You see what happens when you help others.

Chapter 16: Stress Relief

Do a little exercise every day

Exercise can increase or decrease cortisol levels, depending on how intense you exercise. Cortisol levels will rise if you do intense exercise. This is evident shortly after the end of your exercise. This temporary increase is balanced at night. As it coordinates body growth, the short-term increase can be beneficial. It is possible to reduce the cortisol response by regular training.

If an individual is not physically fit, even moderate exercise can increase cortisol levels (Puterman and co., 2011). A person who is physically fit will experience a lower elevation in cortisol levels. Exercise results in lower cortisol levels during the night. Moderate exercise at 40-60% of maximum intensity does not increase cortisol levels, but it also provides lower levels of cortisol in the evenings.

Exercise will lower cortisol levels at night. While intense exercise may temporarily increase cortisol levels, it will decrease over the course of the night.

Indulge in Any Spiritual Pursuit

Cortisol levels can be reduced if you have a spiritual inclination. There are many stresses in life, including illness. Those with a spiritual faith have lower cortisol levels. This was in addition to the projected value due to the cortisol-lowering effect of social support one receives in their groups. Prayer can also be a positive factor in reducing anxiety and depression.

Meditation is another option for those who are spiritually inclined. Joining a support group can be a great way to relieve stress and do acts of kindness.

People with spiritual inclinations, such as those who pray and develop faith, can receive good feedback. Doing acts of kindness can lower cortisol levels.

Try Relaxation Techniques

There are many exercises that can help you relax. Some require mental and passive effort, while others require physical effort. You should choose the ones that you feel most comfortable with and continue to practice them every day. "But, physical activity is important to stress reduction. You don't need to do a lot to reap its benefits," Pick (2018).

Start with deep-breathing exercises. This simple exercise is quick and effective in reducing stress. It can be used anywhere, anytime. Deep breathing exercises were shown to reduce cortisol levels by 50% in middle-aged women. Different relaxation techniques can also reduce cortisol levels.

Massage is another great way to reduce stress levels and cortisol. A weekly massage can help reduce cortisol by 30%. Yoga can also be helpful in managing stress and reducing cortisol. Tai chi is a great way to reduce stress.

Music can reduce cortisol levels, and it can also relax the body. The cortisol levels drop to half their original level if one listens for 30 minutes to music. One test showed that reading is also relaxing. If you have no other options, it is sufficient to maintain silence for 30 minutes. To escape stress and elevated cortisol, make sure to practice these techniques often.

One could use any of many relaxation techniques to lower cortisol levels. These include deep breathing, yoga, massage, music and tai-chi.

Your best self is what you should be doing

It is normal to feel guilt or shame at times in your life. It should not cause negative thinking as this will only increase cortisol levels. An adult group participated in a program that helped them identify and deal with low emotions. The participants saw a 23% reduction in cortisol compared to the 15 non-participating adult group.

You can overcome guilt feelings by addressing the root cause. It might be necessary for you to make some lifestyle changes. Sometimes, it is possible to forgive yourself and solve the problem. This will improve your sense of well-being. Forging stable relationships requires that one learn to forgive others. This is an important part of marriage counseling. Interventions helped couples resolve their conflicts, which resulted in lower cortisol levels.

Resolving your guilt can help increase cortisol levels. This might include making lifestyle changes, learning to forgive others, and forgiving yourself.

Take a break to have fun

This is a great way to reduce cortisol levels. There are many ways you can remain happy. Positive dispositions help lower blood pressure and cortisol. Healthy heart beats are good for the immune system and help to improve and strengthen it.

You will be able to improve your health and have more fun doing things that increase your life satisfaction. This will allow you to control your cortisol. One study showed that laughter can reduce cortisol levels. You should engage in hobbies that increase happiness and prosperity. A group of veterans who started gardening saw a drop in cortisol levels. The control group opted for traditional occupations.

A group of 30 people took up reading, and they experienced a decrease in stress and cortisol. Sometimes, it was possible to reduce stress by spending time outside. However, this is not always true.

Build healthy relationships

The interaction you have with your family members and friends can bring you great joy, but also cause stress. Understanding how cortisol levels fluctuate is essential to determine which one is best for you.

Cortisol in Hair

Cortisol can be found in the hair in very small quantities. The amount of cortisol in the hair will vary depending on where it is located and when it was tested. The results of hair testing are often done and used by researchers to determine the cortisol level.

Reports indicate that children who come from stable families have a significantly lower cortisol level in their hair, which is indicative of a happy, warm family life (Vaghri and co., 2013). They observed that couples who were involved in conflicts experienced a temporary rise in cortisol levels, which then dropped back to their normal levels within a few minutes. They found that cortisol levels returned quickly to normal after a miscommunication when they were able to compare different styles and conflicts.

Support from loved ones can help reduce cortisol levels in stressful situations. The researchers found that men with the support of their female companions had lower cortisol levels when they spoke in public. A second observation was that a close relationship with your partner prior to any activity that increases stress had a positive effect on your blood pressure and heart rate, compared to support from a friend.

Having more family and friends increases happiness and decreases stress. You learn to forgive and you have better emotional stability which leads to good health.

To sum it all, you need to be happy in order to lower cortisol levels. You can achieve this by engaging in a hobby or spending more time outside.

Chapter 17: How to deal with stress at work

There are many factors that influence how much work stress you experience. We put great effort into finding and keeping our job because it is what gives us life. Unfortunately, it is rare to find a job that provides both financial security as well as personal satisfaction. Many problems at work can cause stress, which can lead to poor productivity and lower performance. This can ultimately lead to emotional and physical disorders. A reasonable amount of stress at work can be beneficial. If you're given a task to complete and know that you will be promoted or receive a reward or a promotion, stress can help you stay motivated and focused. Chronic stress can also be caused by increased demands at work, long hours, and other serious problems like lack of recognition from your superiors or coworkers, a lack of meaning in what they are doing, fear about job security, or dissatisfaction with their job. Although we cannot control the environment at work, there are steps that can be taken to lessen stress.

Improve your relationships with coworkers

You can begin by building positive relationships with your coworkers. This allows you to share thoughts, opinions, and feelings with someone with whom you have something in common. You can relieve stress from your workplace and feel calmer. You can take a break from thinking about work and stare at your phone, to start chatting with your coworkers. Having supportive and positive colleagues can help reduce stress levels. Although they may not be able to fix your problems or theirs, having someone to talk with and someone who is willing to listen can make a big difference. You can make a difference by showing empathy and support to your coworkers. This will bring you joy and reduce stress.

Change your focus from your mind towards your body

It is important to shift your focus away from work when things become too stressful. This can be done by taking a break and getting away from stressful situations. Moving around will help you to clear your mind and restore your balance. You can keep stress under control by adding any type of exercise to your daily routine. You can relax your mind and body by dancing, swimming, running, or walking, and it will help you stay focused.

Get good sleep

Stress can lead to insomnia, and if you don't get enough sleep, you will be even more stressed. It is important to get enough sleep, good sleep, and rest. This will help you maintain your emotional balance and increase your productivity. You can improve your quality of sleep by arranging your day so that you get eight hours sleep each night. Avoid stressful situations prior to bedtime. Before you go to sleep, listen to soft music and read. You may be more susceptible to stress if you work shifts. This can affect the quality of your sleeping. You can try to avoid rotating shifts or limit irregular night shifts. This will help you to avoid sleep deprivation.

Take note of what you eat

The importance of food at work is significant. It is crucial to maintain a steady level of blood sugar during work. This can be achieved by eating small, frequent, healthy meals. It will give you energy and help you stay focused. Smoking is a strong stimulant that can increase anxiety and should be avoided. Alcohol is also affected. Alcohol temporarily reduces stress, but can cause anxiety to return as the effects wear off. Do not eat comfort food and increase your intake of omega-3 fat acids to boost your mood.

You need to balance your work and leisure hours

You can cope with stress by finding a balance between your work and family life, your leisure time, and your daily responsibilities. Although this is not an easy task, it can be done if you pay attention even to the smallest, seemingly insignificant things. Running late in the morning can make you unhappy and cause you to be anxious when you arrive at work. You can make a difference by leaving earlier in the morning. This will allow you to start your day more relaxed. Take a break during work hours to chat with colleagues, and then go to lunch. This will allow you to relax and improve your productivity.

Chapter 18: Naturally Boosting Testosterone

Even if the idea of taking testosterone supplements seems unconvincing, it is because we all agree. Low testosterone levels can be corrected by lifestyle changes. Doctors could prescribe testosterone in the form supplements or steroids. However, more knowledgeable doctors would recommend a vacation to let your mind wander and focus on your health. The vicious circle of stress and low levels T hormone will continue until the cycle is broken. It is important to eliminate the major factors that keep you in the low-testosterone loop.

Your doctor will ask about your lifestyle. If he believes in natural T-hormone boosting, he will keep to the following factors:

Sleep as much as you can

It is hard to overstate the benefits of good sleep. This is because it can help you with your overall health, as well as other conditions that may be hindering your ability to function at peak levels. According to a urology professor at George Washington Medical Center, Washington D.C., low testosterone could be due to sleep deprivation. Sleep deprivation can cause adverse effects on nearly all hormones and affect the chemical processes that maintain healthy levels.

No matter what you are doing, sleep should always be your priority. You will see the benefits of sleep, along with healthy eating and a active lifestyle. Many people struggle to fall asleep at their preferred time. If this happens frequently, it is not unusual for many people.

Keep your body healthy

You should bring your Body Mass Index up to a healthy percentile if you are overweight or underweight to maintain your testosterone levels. There have been links between low testosterone levels and unhealthy body weight. Therefore, it is important to maintain a healthy body weight.

Keep active!

Although we don't recommend you become a bodybuilder or any other type of professional, we suggest that you add some activities to your otherwise boring lifestyle. Researchers have found that testosterone is released according to the body's needs. Your testosterone levels may drop if you spend a lot of time sitting down or lying down, as your body does not require as much testosterone.

Begin slow, then pick up speed as you go. Here are some activities you might consider starting:

* Brisk walking for 15-20 minutes per day. Once you feel comfortable with the pace and distance, you can increase the speed or time.

* Strength training is a great way to increase testosterone levels in your brain.

To burn fat and build muscle mass, you'll need to use your body weight. However, the T hormone is required for optimal functioning. Your adrenal glands will release it when your brain sends a message. This is the best way to get your body to produce more testosterone.

* Weight training is another method to increase testosterone. You can start slowly and gradually increase your weight. Working with a certified trainer is a great way to make sure you have proper form and posture while working out.

Don't overdo it. This could lead to injuries and lower testosterone, as can be seen with endurance athletes.

Do not allow stress to overwhelm you

It sounds strange, but it is true when stress can overwhelm and exhaust you. Stress is the greatest problem of our time. Being under constant stress can cause our bodies to release cortisol, a stress hormone that further aggrave situations.

The body has a hard time releasing testosterone when it is under stress. You will need to find ways to deal with the stress at work. Take, for example:

It is possible to cut down on the hours you work at night, even though it sounds impossible. You can ensure your health by finishing work before midnight, and moving on to the next task. It is recommended that you work less than 10 hours per day to maintain your health.

* Work and exercise require a certain level of commitment. Both are essential to your survival. However, you can spend an hour every day doing something that is not related to one of them.

Which medicines are you currently taking?

You might need to take medication that is likely to lower your testosterone levels if you have chronic illnesses. Your testosterone levels may also be affected if you are an athlete, bodybuilder, or any other type of person who needs to maintain your performance. To make a difference, you don't have to stop taking your medications. Instead, you should ask your doctor to rule out the possibility and find a way to increase your testosterone without disrupting your daily life.

Stop adding to your diet

If you want to boost your testosterone levels, this is the most important lesson you should learn. There will be many temptations. From media ads to online advertisements, friends and acquaintances may swear by XYZ to instantly increase testosterone levels. Stop falling for the temptations of a supplement. Supplements can ruin your self-confidence and make you believe they are effective. They will then disappoint you.

DHEA, a hormone that can convert itself into testosterone, is naturally produced by our bodies. DHEA supplements can be sold to those with low testosterone. However, these products don't make any difference in reality. To date, there has not been any substantiated evidence that DHEA supplements are effective.

The body produces testosterone under certain conditions. If these conditions are not met, the body will not produce the optimal levels. This is why it is important to have faith in your body's ability to secrete sufficient T hormones. Follow the above guidelines. While you can refer to many health professionals, the fundamental principles must be followed.

Chapter 19: The 5 Stages of Sleep

Traditional wisdom has five stages to fall asleep. These stages include stages one through four, and REM sleep. Rapid Eye Movement is also known as REM. This is the most important part of your sleep. These stages are progressive and you will go through them from 1 to 4. Then, you'll enter the dreaming stage which is responsible for your body, mind, and energy levels. While the standard sleep cycle lasts approximately 90 minutes, each person's exact time will vary. Our brains move through various stages during sleep cycles, resulting in a dynamic performance.

These stages are progressively occurring throughout the night. However, they all change throughout the night.

This is a more detailed breakdown of each stage, and how it affects your sleep cycle.

Stage 1:

This is often referred to by the stage when you drift in and out of sleep, depending on how tired you are. After a long day, your body activity slows down and you can be woken up quickly. Twitching can be a common symptom during this stage and can even cause a falling sensation in your body. This stage is not very helpful for us. It is used as a portal into our sleep state.

Stage 2

Stage two is when things get "moving" with respect to sleep production. This stage is when our brain frequencies and eye movements slow down. There are bursts in brain waves during the second stage. These brain waves bursts are called sleeping spindles. These waves are technically called sigma waves and have a frequency of twelve to fourteen.

K-complexes, another amazing phenomenon, can be seen at this stage. These complexes are fascinating to say the very least. These complexes have short negative high voltage peaks that are followed by a more positive complex. This completes the K-complexes with another negative peak. Each complex lasts approximately one to two minutes.

This stage of sleep protects our sleeping cycle. This stage is where our circadian rhythm becomes less efficient. This stage is where stimulus recognition from outside becomes suppressed. It also helps with the consolidation of memories and experiences, as well as the processing important information that has been collected through the subconscious processing system.

Stage 3

Stage three results from the slowing down of our sleep during preparation for your first two sleep cycles. This stage is also known as deep sleep, or slow wave sleep. Our environment becomes less responsive throughout this stage. Our awareness shifts to sleeping, and our environment becomes less responsive. This blocking out of time is more common in the first half our sleep cycle.

The Stage 3 stage is responsible for approximately 15% to 20% of our sleep time during our normal sleeping patterns.

Stage two sleep spindles still occur, but at a much lower frequency. This stage is when the brain produces delta waves, which emit a very low frequency than other stages of sleep. The frequency of delta brain waves can range from half a Hertz to four hertz.

Because they operate within the same frequency, stages three and four are closely connected. Stage three, however, is where the body's lowest functioning stage. This stage of sleep is when your breathing and brain temperature are the lowest.

You will also experience your lowest blood pressure and heart rate at this time. The third stage is where we most often enter our dreams, but without generating REM. These dreams are often dull and hazy in comparison to the vivid and dynamic dreams we experience during our REM sleep cycle.

Stage three is where you'll experience night terrors and sleep walking. This is the stage of sleep your body is experiencing if you have ever had little sleep or woke up feeling groggy. Your sleeping cycle will have less stage three activity the older you become. Children tend to sleep longer than adults and seniors get very little or no stage three sleep.

Stage 4

The stage four stage is where the brain operates at lower frequencies than the higher frequency flux that occurs frequently in stage three. The stage has no eye movement or body movement.

Stage four can be described as the calm before the storm, which is about to enter the most important stage in sleep.

Officially, Stage 4 is a variant on stage 3. However, these stages are different in terms stability and frequency.

Stage 5: REM

The magic happens in Stage 5. This stage of sleep is very dynamic but also makes us feel awake, rested, and alert the next morning. The REM sleep cycles usually last between ninety and one hundred and twenty minutes. It's responsible in total for between one and a quarter of your adult sleeping hours. Our REM sleep appears to decline over time, just like in stage 3. Infants can sleep in REM for up to 80% of their 14-17 hours of sleep. This is a lot of dreaming!

REM sleep is the main driving force in the second half our sleeping cycle. Each cycle that we are asleep allows us to dive deeper in to REM. If you have ever had to stop sleeping, it is because your hours before waking are filled with REM.

Rapid Eye Movement (REM) is a stage in sleep where our minds run wild. While our eyes are closed, we may experience "random" or sporadic eye movements. The only way to determine the stage of sleep you are in is by using electrooculography (also known as EOG).

Experts were able to determine that the eye movement shifts from a tonic state to a phasic. However, no one has yet to explain why. My belief is that rapid eye movements stimulate brain activity via the same communication channels responsible for brain interactions with stories. Although there isn't any scientific evidence to support our dreams, brain activity studies have provided more insight into what happens to the brain when we dream.

It is possible that dreaming and REM sleeping are not dependent. Other research suggests that we might not be dreaming. Subliminal images are processed by our subconscious during transitions into waking state. Our dreams could be the result of subliminal language processing.

There is currently no research available that can help us understand this type of information processing. Eugen Tarnow suggested that this type of processing could be the compilation and processing experiences into long-term support for the experience that is common to all major belief systems. This theory is supported by the fact that children younger than 5 years old are often asleep. This correlates with research showing that belief systems are largely formed in the first year of life.

Dreaming, in other words is the language of your subconscious that uses the power of story to create a dynamic processing system of your belief system and its reactions. This is what likely causes the regeneration of your body, and all cells within it.

REM can be described as a low-amplitude combination of brain frequencies that reflect our brain processes while we are awake. It includes beta, alpha, and theta waves. These are used when we experience focus and flow. This paradoxical style of sleep causes our brain to consume more oxygen and energy than usual when we are facing complex or challenging problems.

When we are in REM sleep, our breathing experiences a similar situation to when we see. As our brain activity increases, our heart rate and blood pressure increase, our breathing changes from slow and steady to fast and irregular.

But there is one thing that distinguishes our dreaming from our waking states. During REM, our physical body becomes completely deactivated, and our body becomes paralyzed. Atonia is the result of brain impulses that stimulate muscle movement being "disconnected" to your muscles. The powerful stimulations during

REM sleep can cause the body to be disconnected. This is thought to be an preventative measure to protect our body while our minds are engaged in "muscle moving" activities. If our brain does not receive enough REM during sleep, it will compensate by absorbing it at the fastest possible time.

As we learn new skills, spatial memory is strengthened during this stage of sleep. After a long day of learning, people often feel tired. These situations can cause us to experience more REM sleep than normal.

We often wake up during our sleep cycle in short bursts lasting only a few seconds. These situations are not often remembered. If the events trigger our wakefulness, it can take a whole sleeping cycle to fall asleep again. It is difficult to fall asleep if you wake up during the night.

Although there is still much to be learned about REM, we do have a good understanding of how it works in the past.

This stage is essential for our ability to function. How much REM sleep we get directly affects how recharged and refreshed we feel when the day ends.

Chapter 20: Supplements that Really Work

There are many supplements that can help with chronic fatigue. Many also work quickly as an energy booster. These supplements will make you feel better quickly. You should inform your doctor about any supplement or pill you take. Natural supplements can interact with prescription and over-the-counter medications. Make sure your doctor is aware of any changes in your daily routine.

Supplement #1 Glycine

It is an amino supplement, which can often improve cognitive performance in just one or two doses. Although it is found in many foods, the supplement will give you an additional boost. This supplement can help you sleep better. It is recommended to take three grams of the supplement, which is not expensive.

Supplement #2 Theanine

It can also be found in green tea as an amino acid. This amino acid is great for helping you sleep but it shouldn't be mistaken for a sedative. It improves your sleep quality and makes you feel more rested when you wake up each morning. It is recommended to take 150 to 200 mgs of it half an hour before bed if you are looking to improve your sleep quality. You will feel refreshed enough to fight your chronic fatigue the next day. It's also a cheap supplement that you can easily add to your daily routine.

Supplement #3 Rhodiola Rosaa

This is an adoptigen because it can help you desensitize to stressful events before they happen. It is great for treating metabolic burnout and mild depression. It can help you maintain healthy levels of serotonin, which will improve your mood and hormones. You should use it every day at 150 mg. You will need to ensure that they are one percent salidrosidie and three percent rosavins.

Supplement #4 Creatine

It is a dietary supplement which will help promote energy and counter fatigue from over exertion. It is known to increase muscle mass and help prevent fatigue. Although many doctors believe it is safe to use for the long-term, you should still consult your doctor. There are some issues with this medicine.

Supplement #5 Glucose

You might consider glucose as a stimulant. You can use it to increase your performance and to maintain your energy levels. You can add glucose to water. Usually, you can drink between twenty and forty grams of glucose during a workout. Your doctor will advise you how to take it depending on your type of chronic fatigue. It can be safely added to your diet.

Supplement #6 Melatonin

You may not get the sleep you want or need if you are having trouble sleeping due to fatigue. Melatonin has been shown to improve quality and quantity of sleep. It can help you get up in the morning feeling refreshed so you can get your day started on the right foot. It will reduce fatigue over time. Your body might not want to go to sleep if there is too much light. Melatonin may be able help.

Supplement #7 Vitamin C

If you are suffering from fatigue, vitamin C is a must. You can feel even more fatigue if you don't have enough vitamin C. Vitamin C can prevent fatigue from various infections, which can lead to chronic fatigue. Vitamin C can increase your body's ability to absorb iron from the digestive track. This can reduce fatigue and anemia which can lead to fatigue. You are more likely to develop allergies and fatigue if you don't have enough vitamin C.

Supplement #8 Vitamin E

Vitamin E can also be very helpful if you are suffering from fatigue. This is because Vitamin E helps to boost your immune system, which can help keep fatigue away. Vitamin E is an antioxidant that will protect your cells and can prevent anemia. Vitamin E can be helpful for people with vitamin E deficiency. Vitamin E can also be used in conjunction with prescription and over-the-counter medications.

Supplement #9 Zinc

Zinc can be very important in combating fatigue. It can also help to increase muscle strength and endurance. Zinc can improve immune function and reduce fatigue. Zinc can also aid in digestion and metabolism. Zinc can be obtained from food, but it can often prove difficult to obtain enough. Zinc can be found in whole grain wheat bran and pumpkin seeds as well as wheat germ. However, if you're deficient in zinc, it might not be enough. Supplement #10 Potassium

It is common to have potassium deficiencies. However, you will find that potassium can help increase your energy and vitality. It can reduce fatigue and muscular weakness, as well as help with chronic fatigue. It can restore energy and prevent your muscles from aching, which many people feel when they are suffering from chronic fatigue. It can also help maintain a healthy heart beat and nervous system function.

Supplement #11 Calcium

Chronic fatigue can lead to stress. Calcium can help reduce that stress as well as the fatigue. Calcium can reduce anxiety, nervous tension, emotional upset, and other symptoms. Low calcium levels can lead to mood swings, fatigue, muscle irritability, and cramps. Calcium is an essential part of your diet and can be easily added to your daily routine with minimal to no side effects. You should consult your doctor before you add it to your daily routine.

Supplement #12 Maca Root

Maca root may be a good option for chronic fatigue. Maca root regulates cortisol, which can help with anxiety and stress. It may also improve blood sugar levels. It may help with adrenal fatigue.

Supplement #13 Licorice Root

Supplements can be taken with licorice root. It supports adrenal gland fatigue and helps with chronic fatigue. Although you can drink licorice root tea it may not be as effective as the supplement and the taste might not be as appealing. You can ask your doctor before you add licorice root supplement to your daily routine. It can increase your endurance and help you fight fatigue throughout the day. It has been shown to increase hormone production, which can help many people. You should know that licorice root can increase blood pressure when used as a supplement. Your doctor must also be informed before you include it in your daily routine.

Chapter 21: Swap Your Joe For A Cup O' Green Tea

Do you find yourself one of those people who just has to have a cup every morning? Do you feel like a zombie until your mandatory cup of coffee is finished? You are. You want to increase your energy, right? I was that zombie once. Before I had my first cup, my kids couldn't speak a word to me. I was tempted to drink four to five cups of coffee before running off to work. But my concern about my blood pressure and skyrocketing blood sugar overpowered that desire. What if there was a beverage you could have that provides more energy than coffee and can even help you lose weight? It sounds too good to be true! It's not true! After perusing a variety of fitness magazines, I made a decision: green tea was the best. It was a huge decision for me to switch to green tea from coffee.

When I was twelve years of age, I started to take sips from my mom's cup of coffee.

After my senior year in high school, I began to make my own coffee. It was difficult to break my dependency on coffee. What could possibly compare to my coffee-loving green tea leaves? It turned out that green tea exceeded all my expectations.

Both green teas and coffee are rich in antioxidants. However, green tea has the antioxidant catechin. Research on catechins has shown that they play a protective role in preventing heart disease, type 1 diabetes, and obesity. Although it may be associated with preventing certain types, more research is needed to confirm this theory.

Prozac may be an option for you if you suffer from anxiety problems that can also cause major energy loss. Theanine is a unique amino acid found in green tea that acts as a natural relaxant. It also has significant anti-anxiety benefits. Green tea drinkers have a higher concentration than coffee-drinkers.

As an aside, oolong and black teas can be substituted for coffee. Both green and black teas are made from the Camellia Sinesis plant. What the leaves were cooked is what makes the difference between the three types of teas. The green tea is the least processed, while the other two have significantly more fermented leaf. The best form of energy is green tea, so it's worth choosing this one over the others.

Stay tuned if you are still skeptical about green tea's benefits for energy and weight loss. The most convincing factor in green tea is the inclusion of EGCG. EGCG (epicatechin galate) is a catechin polyphenol and is the most extensively researched component of green tea. Research has shown that green tea contains EGCG, which can help speed up metabolism. In a recent study, the American Journal of Clinical Nutrition found that EGCG and caffeine can increase your metabolism by approximately 4%

over 24 hours. Ten men were included in the study. Half of them received caffeine only, and the other half were given both 50 mgs of caffeine and 90 mgs of EGCG. Men who had EGCG and caffeine combined showed a 4% increase in metabolism. Those who only consumed caffeine alone did not show any change. EGCG has been shown to reduce the absorption and absorption of fats. This is a clear benefit for weight loss.

Green tea has approximately a third of caffeine as coffee. You can have up to five cups of green tea per day. If you have an existing problem with caffeine, it is unlikely that you will experience any side effects. When it comes to caffeine, three cups of green tea are equal to one cup coffee. If you substitute your morning coffee with three cups of green tea, you will get the same caffeine intake but three times more energy. That's a fantastic deal, if ever there was one!

These are some things you should keep in mind when switching from coffee to green-tea. You should be aware that green tea is acidic and you may need to pay attention to how your body reacts to it, particularly if you have had acid-related problems in the past. Green tea might not be suitable for those with acid reflux. You shouldn't have any unpleasant side effects if you drink it in small amounts and take an off-the-shelf or prescribed antacid medication. You can also switch to LoHan, an all-natural sugar replacement, if you want to sweeten your morning drink. The simple fact that green tea is lower in calories than coffee is due to the fact that many people like to add flavorful items to their coffee. These sweets can lead to high caloric costs over the long-term. You can easily add a lot of calories to your coffee with sugar, coffee-mate, and other artificial flavors to make it more delicious. These are the main reasons tea drinkers avoid sweeteners. Natural sugar substitutes are clearly better than artificial sweeteners like Splenda. These sweeteners, while being lower in calories and more nutritious than table sugar, can actually be harmful to the body. Studies have shown that artificial sweeteners may increase your risk of certain types and forms of cancer.

Don't think about buying a bottled green tea drink to sip on the way to work. You need to stop! These products should not be on your shopping cart. The fact that green tea extracts have many health benefits is evident to companies that make bottled beverages. Snapple, which markets green tea extracts, has become more aware of these health benefits and has started to market Snapple drinks. Although they may contain some green tea extracts, the beverages are dominated by sugar and artificial flavors. While you may think you are drinking a healthy beverage, the sugar and artificial flavorings in these beverages can make it more unhealthy. It is best to make your own green tea. You will get the best results if you use the actual tea leaves and not the bags that come with the tea bags. However, it is better than buying expensive bottled tea. You can sweeten your tea with a little bit of natural sugar substitute, but not too much. Natural alternatives are strong and you won't usually need much. You can add some lime or lemon to give it an extra flavor. As long as your acid-related issues are not a problem, you can do so. Acid is a natural component of citrus fruits.

Chapter 22: 7 Things You can Do to Get Rid of Fatigue

If you feel constantly tired and slow, despite the fact that you may be getting enough sleep during the night, then you could be among millions of people who have given up on the quality of their lives to constant fatigue. You can easily get rid of fatigue in some simple ways.

There are many reasons you feel fatigued. Knowing how to identify these issues can help you eliminate your fatigue. These are some things you might find useful in fighting tiredness.

1. Limit your evening sleep to 15 to 45 minutes. If you sleep longer than this, you may feel tired and drowsy. You may feel drowsy if you sleep more than you should.

2. Rest and get up. Your wake-up timer should be set to the exact time you need to get up. You may feel tired if you delay your waking hours. To ensure a good

night's sleep, you can clean up before going to bed.

3. Eliminated caffeine. Although it might cause you to be more alert after taking it, the effects of caffeine can make you feel even more tired. To avoid being anxious at night, you should also avoid caffeine for several hours before going to bed.

4. Move your body. The main reason for tiredness is a lack of exercise. In this way, if you are looking to get rid of fatigue, start a new lifestyle and do some work out. You can kick start your day by doing a 30-minute cardio exercise before breakfast.

5. Regular water intake is a must. Constant tiredness can also be caused by dry skin. Make sure you drink enough water to keep your body hydrated. Your body will be in a dynamic state if you have enough water and other fluids. Caffeinated drinks can give you an instant boost of energy, but the effects may last for several hours.

6. Do not let worry take over your life. One of the main causes of many medical problems that people experience is stress. If you feel tired and slow, it is time to get some push. To get rid of stress, go swimming. Do it consistently. Take control of your time. Avoid lingering. This will allow you to concentrate on the best way to get rid of fatigue.

7. Pay attention to your weight. If you're overweight or underweight you might feel constantly tired. If you're overweight or large, your body will need to work harder to perform basic exercises. This can lead to feelings of tiredness. You may feel fatigued if you lack muscle quality. To avoid fatigue, you should maintain a normal weight.

Chapter 23: Why is it Raw?

Many people wonder why raw food is better than cooked food. Most people are comfortable with eating cooked food, and very few have been raised on raw food.

Although the effects of cooking on food are not well understood, they can have serious consequences. These were highlighted by Professor Rosalind Graham in an article published for the UK Fruitfest newsletter.

Raw is the best!

By Professor Rozalind Graham

Carbohydrates and Heat: The Effects

Dextrin is formed when starches are cooked in water or steam. This is a simpler carbohydrate than starch. Cooked starches can still be difficult to digest because of hydrolysis, which occurs when they are heated in water or steam. These water-saturated foods make the digestive enzyme amylase, or ptyalin, ineffective.

Amylase is used for the conversion of polysaccharides to disaccharides. If this is not possible, the carbohydrates ferment in your gut and produce acetic acid (vinegar), various alcoholics, and carbon dioxide gas. Acetic acid can be used to stimulate the thyroid gland and leach phosphorous from the body. The adrenal glands' ability to function properly is affected if phosphorus levels are low.

This can lead to headaches, throat congestion and mucous production as well as pains in the heart and body. When starches are exposed to heat directly, they become caramalized and can lead to the formation of harmful substances known as carcinogenic.

The Heat Effects on Proteins

Heat is a dangerous habit that can make food unusable.

The cooking process creates enzyme-resistant bonds between amino acid chains, making them resistant to digestion.

The long chains of amino acid, also known as peptides can penetrate the gut wall, causing havoc in the system. This stimulates prostaglandin activity, which in turn triggers the auto immune response, leading to conditions such as arthritis and gout.

Sulphur is an important disinfecting ingredient in human nutrition. Sulphur is found in both the amino acids Cystine (and Methionine) The body cannot use the inorganic, incomplete molecule of sulphur that is formed when it is heated in the presence water. Although cystine is vital for the formation red corpuscles, it is rendered ineffective once the sulphur is gone.

Body serum, haemoglobin, and tissue all contain methionine. It is also unusable because of the loss of its sulfur due to cooking.

Heat and Fats

Heating fats poses greater health risks than any other nutrients, as they are carcinogenic. Because fats cannot be emulsified, heat makes them non-assimilable.

They can then become carcinogenic by allowing the body to release poisons that are not contained in its fluids. This has serious implications for the overall health of the organism as fats are processed through the lymphatic system.

Additionally, once temperatures rise to 350 degrees (the temperature for cooking and frying), fats start to break down and their vitamins and minerals become unusable. The cooking process renders almost all fat-soluble vitamins in fatty foods useless.

Fats are the hardest nutrients to digest. High-fat foods can cause the food bolus to remain longer in the stomach and may lead to fermentation of carbohydrates or the depletion of proteins.

This is because fat tends to cover the food particles, making it difficult for enzymes and digestive juices to penetrate.

Additionally, cooked fats can also coat the lining and prevent the secretion digestive juices from being released.

Acroleic acid, a poisonous carcinogen that forms when fats are cooked, is formed by heat on glycerol. Acrolein, a gas emitted during cooking, can cause cancer in the lungs. This has been demonstrated by people who work in deep-frying food production.

Frying is one of the most unhealthy forms of cooking. Repeated use of the same oil (as is common in deep fat frying) is also dangerous.

It is important that you realize that all foods contain fats to some extent and all cooked foods are carcinogenic.

After cooked fats are absorbed into bloodstream, they cause blood to become sticky. This can lead to thrombosis or a stroke.

Conclusion

To quickly regain energy, you must change your lifestyle. You will be glad that you took the initiative to take action in the first place. Every physical action you take increases your metabolism, making it easier to find more energy. It is true that energy creates more energy.

It is also important to drink enough water. How can you help your muscles fight fatigue if they aren't getting enough water? Your mind is full of negative thoughts, how can you expect your body to want to exercise? It is time to shift gears. Give your body the right food, enough water, and enough exercise.

When I felt low in energy, I realized that I didn't enjoy any type of sport and needed to find something that I enjoyed. I chose dancing. I used my iPad to watch videos and then did Zumba. After making sure I was properly dressed and had not eaten, I began to do it twice daily and noticed a huge increase in my energy levels. How come? Energy is energy. You will be more successful if you choose an activity you love and not try to avoid it. You will see a difference in your life if you start to do these activities regularly.

These methods are great for those who have been through bad experiences or become sedentary and have fallen into a rut. It is important to determine if there are any medical reasons for your lack of energy. This will give you the assurance that nothing is wrong and can help you feel better. You can then use your energy to increase your energy, sleep like a baby, and help your body heal itself.

Some people blame their age. Some blame their weight or inactivity on life. It's never too late for you to make a change and stand out. Even if you start small, you'll soon discover that these hobbies are very enjoyable and that the fresh air and natural beauty of nature makes you more positive about life. You can take a walk in the forest, or on a beach in spring. Or you can go for a sunset stroll. The meditation and relaxation techniques in this book will help you incorporate these activities into your daily life. You will see energy return almost immediately if you do this. All it needed was you to let go of negativity and get moving. Jump rope can be a lot of fun with kids. Children are a great way to get your energy up. You might find it helpful to look after the children of a neighbor. This will help you see where your energy is going and allow you to restore your energy. This is the great thing about being around kids. They don't allow you to make the same excuses. They show you how you can energize yourself again and feel great. Even if you are only taking the dog for a walk, having a pet can help boost your energy levels. Don't kid yourself. You can get your energy back quickly by walking with your dog and lose your fatigue.

www.ingramcontent.com/pod-product-compliance
Lightning Source LLC
Chambersburg PA
CBHW070913080526
44589CB00013B/1280